GET THE SKINNY

ANSWERS TO 45 FREQUENTLY ASKED HEALTH & FITNESS QUESTIONS

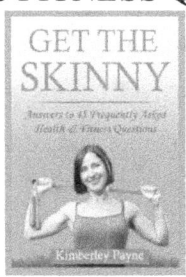

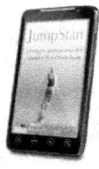 **Your Free Gift**

JumpStart – Launch your journey to improve physical and spiritual fitness

Want to make simple changes to improve spiritual and physical health? Discover a daily, specific program to create a routine.

Visit https://www.kimberleypayne.com/jumpstart/

Contents

Introduction

When I worked full-time as a personal trainer, I fielded many questions from my clients asking for clarification on something they recently read or heard. Usually, it was a myth that had surfaced as truth and my client would wonder about its legitimacy.

This book was born out of those questions. It frustrates me that the health and fitness industry is pumping out false claims and confusing honest people who are just looking to be fit and healthy.

Get the Skinny – Answers to 45 Frequently Asked Health & Fitness Questions was first shared over the "airwaves" on HopeStreamRadio, hopestreamradio.com then transcribed into blog posts on my website under the category of Fit Tips www.kimberleypayne.com/category/fit-tip.

I've researched 45 frequently asked questions and collected them together here.

If you have a question that was not addressed here or want to debunk a myth, I'd love to hear from you!

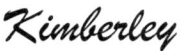

Does fat free mean calorie free?

When I sat down to eat a few cookies I didn't intend to eat ALL the cookies.

"No matter," I thought. "They're low fat."

But that's where they get you. Low fat does not mean calorie free.

I had assumed because they were low fat I could eat double the amount I would normally eat. But most food companies know that when they take out the fat they must replace it with something. And that something is usually sugar. So they load up the item with the sweet stuff to compensate for the lack of flavour from the loss of fat.

You may think you're doing well in reducing your fat intake only to discover that you're actually taking in more calories at each sitting.

Dried fruits are another culprit. Although they are low-fat snacks that are great source of energy and iron beware how many you munch on as they are high in calories.

If you want to lower your fat intake, choosing less processed or prepared foods will be your best bet.

When a food is naturally low fat, the manufacturers don't need to boost flavour with adding calories.

So instead of eating an entire box of Snackwells, next time I'll opt for one or two full fat cookies and a banana on the side.

Is any exercise better than none?

When I worked as a personal trainer, the number one complaint from my clients was that they didn't have time to exercise.

Truthfully, who has time? We're all very busy with work, family, volunteer commitments, household chores, etc.

Adding 3 hours to spend at the gym just doesn't realistically fit into our schedules.

The good news? It doesn't have to.

Any exercise is better than none.

Taking three 10-minute walks each day will do the job to improve health. Many workplaces allow for a morning and afternoon break plus time for lunch. This is perfect for taking 10 of the 15 minutes to march on the spot behind closed doors, or walk up and down the stairwell, or take a brisk walk outside.

Exercise means active living. It all adds up.

The goal is to take advantage of the small opportunities throughout the day to move your body.

Speaking of which, I'm due to take a break right now. I think I'll go crank the music and dance around my home office for ten minutes.

Does low intensity exercise promote weight loss?

You may be surprised to learn that although I'm a health and fitness enthusiast I actually hate to run.

Walking I love, but running is torture.

I remember working with a client who enjoyed running and had a personal goal to complete a 5K race. She wanted me to join her. Being the good personal trainer I was I ran beside her in the race hating every last second of it.

I never experienced that "runner's high" many runners claim exists. Personally I would much rather walk 10 kilometres than run five.

And truth be told, that's okay. Low intensity exercise (such as walking) will help promote weight loss just like any high intensity workout.

The only difference is the amount of time involved.

The most important factor for losing body fat is the total calories burned, regardless of the rate at which they are burned.

I do have to walk further than I'd have to run but I'm okay with that.

The added benefit for me is that I don't tire as quickly and I'm not prone to the same injuries (especially knee problems) that high-intensity exercises may cause.

Is stretching important?

Can you touch your toes? Go ahead, try it now. See if you can touch your toes. If you can, that's fantastic—good for you. If you're like the majority of us who can't, don't fret.

Degrees of flexibility vary widely among people and even among different muscles and joints. Everyone's flexibility is different. The wonderful thing about stretching is that it can be improved no matter what your age or stage of fitness. The more frequently and regularly you stretch, the more flexible you'll become.

Strength and endurance exercises tend to shorten our muscles and reduce elasticity. In order to improve flexibility, we need to incorporate slow, gentle stretching exercises into our daily routine. And it's important to work at improving it. Like many things you must use it or lose it.

Stretching provides relief from muscle tension and stiffness, improves muscle imbalances, and decreases your risk of injury. Keeping flexible helps with quality of life. Just think about simple things like getting in and out of your car, carrying and putting away groceries, or tying your shoes.

And did you know that stretching benefits your mind as well as your body? When done in a slow and focused manner, stretching can be an excellent way to melt tension and reduce stress. The more frequently and regularly you stretch, the more flexible you'll remain as you age. Once you get into the habit of regularly stretching and start noticing progress, you'll be more motivated to continue.

I challenge you to work on your flexibility and touch your toes by this time next year.

Should I reward every success?

January is typically the month that most people make resolutions and set goals. By the end of February, many people fail to meet or even forget these very goals. By March, we're back to old habits.

As an experienced personal trainer, I'd work with clients to set SMART goals because who'd want to set dumb ones, right? We worked together to choose a long-term goal and then break it down into manageable pieces and weekly targets.

For example, one client wanted to lose 20 pounds by her son's wedding in 3 months. This was realistic and gave her a goal of 1.5 pounds per week.

As we progressed, her problem wasn't in losing the weight but in celebrating her loss up to that point. At five pounds lost she lamented that she still had 15 pounds to go. I had to repeatedly remind her to reward her success.

I suggested she buy herself some nice jewellery to wear at the wedding, take a bubble bath to sooth achy muscles and distress, and take the luxury to call a friend that she hadn't talked to in a while. The important thing was that she needed to reward the success that she had achieved up to that point.

Rewarding your success, no matter how small is positive reinforcement and sets you up to continue on the path to achieve the larger, longer-term goals.

Does muscle change into fat when I stop exercising?

Have you ever seen a photo of a football player who, in his glory days of high school, was pure muscle but then years later his muscles appeared to have morphed into a padding of fat? Maybe you thought, as I once had, that because he stopped weight lifting his muscles changed to fat?

Thankfully this is not true. Muscle and fat are two different types of tissue; you simply cannot turn one into another. The bulk of your fat sits right under your skin, on top of your muscle.

You can increase your muscle mass, and you can decrease your body fat, but one does not directly affect the other. Muscle is what dictates our metabolism so the more muscle we have the more calories we will burn. If you stop strength training your muscles will shrink somewhat. If we start losing muscle our metabolism starts to slow down and we increase body fat. That is why strength training is so important to our everyday routine.

Also, people who exercise regularly tend to eat quite a bit more food than people who maintain a relatively healthy body weight without exercising. Once you stop exercising though, you instantly lose the need for the calories used during your workouts, which is often quite significant. If you don't decrease your food intake when you stop training the extra calories that you would normally have burned up in activity will turn into fat.

So if our football player had kept up with a strength training routine and kept an eye on his food intake he could fare much better in his before and after photos.

Is cutting calories good for long-term weight loss?

Have you ever tried a cabbage-soup only diet? I remember trying this as a teenager and I only lasted two days. But it was probably one of the more successful diet attempts I'd tried.

Cutting calorie intake alone to lose weight is not a good option for the long-term. Generally it's too hard to maintain and you end up gaining back any weight lost.

To effectively lose weight, a healthy lifestyle change includes reducing calories and following a regular activity plan. Exercise burns calories, speeds metabolism, and helps offset the dreaded "plateaus" at which weight loss slows down or stops temporarily.

A large amount of exercise is needed to lose weight without reducing calories, and combining more exercise with less food helps avoid the loss of lean body mass and lowered metabolic rate that occurs with dieting alone.

In addition, a friend of mine told me that when she commits to an exercise plan she feels healthier and this in turn makes her want to eat healthier.

This can also work in reverse. When we're not active we may feel less inclined to choose healthier food options which make us feel bad about ourselves and so we turn to comfort food to soothe ourselves and it becomes a vicious cycle.

Combining an activity plan with cutting food calories is the most effective way to lose weight.

Is warming up the same as stretching?

Years ago when I joined a weekend softball team, I remember the coach instructing us to warm up and then proceeded to lead us through a number of stretches. Looking back now, I cringe at the thought of going through flexibility exercises without first warming up my muscles with some light movements to increase blood flow and heart rate.

Unfortunately even today some people think that warming up and stretching are synonymous. They are not. Stretching a muscle does not warm it. In fact, trying to stretch a cold muscle can lead to injury and is dangerous since muscles have less elasticity when cold.

Stretching and warming up are two different processes. Stretching involves lengthening your muscles whereas warming up means you're elevating your core body temperature and getting blood flowing to the muscles and increasing their temperature. Warmed up muscles stretch better.

First, warm up with a cardiovascular activity such as walking, jumping jacks, or dancing around and then stretch.

Had my softball coach led us through walking the bases or marching on the spot first before stretching we may have made it to the big leagues.

Is the number on the scale a good indication of health?

Have you ever been to the doctor's office and he's asked you to get on the weigh scale? If you're anything like me you remove your shoes first. And then your socks and jewellery. And depending on how modest you are the rest of your clothes. The scale is inevitably 7 pounds heavier than what you were only an hour ago at home. It's distressing and disheartening.

On the other hand, have you ever been at a friend's home and during a visit to the washroom you jump on the scale to "just see". Oh joy, if it's even 1/2 a pound lower than your own scale. You bound out of the bathroom with a grin on your face ready now to accept that second slice of banana bread. Although I'm sure many of us do it, we really shouldn't put so much weight into what the weight on the scale is (pun intended).

The weight on a scale does not indicate your overall health. Your weight is the sum total of your bones, organs, fat, muscles, and other tissue. You can't change the part of your body that is bones, tissues and organs, but you can change the ratio of fat to muscle with good training and proper diet.

Body composition (fat compared to lean body mass) is more important. Two people can weigh exactly the same on a scale and yet be tremendously different in body composition. Since muscle weighs more than fat, the scale weight can be deceiving. For many people, getting on the scale is difficult. But if you focus on body composition, the struggle can be a little bit more tolerable. Weight can fluctuate from day to day, but pay more attention to how you feel and how your clothes fit.

Do crash diets work?

When I was a teenager I toyed with every fad diet out there. Although I wasn't that overweight, I always felt self-conscious about not being skinny. I tried the Grapefruit Diet, Cabbage Soup Diet, and Lemonade Diet. Have you ever tried these diets?

The Grapefruit Diet, also known as the "Hollywood Diet" is based on the claim that grapefruit contains certain enzymes that, when eaten before other foods, helps burn off fat. Sorry, but grapefruit doesn't burn fat. It may be that the water in grapefruit helps you feel full, and then you eat less. But if you're hoping that grapefruit will melt fat, you're going to be disappointed.

The Cabbage-Soup diet isn't much better. It's sometimes referred to as the "Mayo Clinic Diet," or the "Sacred Heart Hospital Diet". A part of this diet plan is to eat cabbage soup, every day and several times a day. But before you stock up on cabbage, know that this crash diet won't help you in the long run, and it doesn't give your body the nutrients it needs to stay healthy.

The Lemonade Diet, also called the "Master Cleanse", is a liquid-only diet consisting of three things: a lemonade-like beverage, salt-water drink, and herbal laxative tea. But again, it's a crash diet that won't make a positive difference in the longer term.

Trying to lose 10 pounds in 10 days isn't healthy. Because you're getting so few calories, you'll probably lose weight. But the weight lost is mainly muscle mass and water, not excess body fat. And you're likely to gain the weight right back.

These crash diets don't include exercise, and working out at high levels isn't a great idea on such a low-calorie diet. Your body just won't have enough energy for exercise. A diet program like these mentioned restricts calories to fewer than 1200 per day which is ineffective and unsafe.

For lasting results, it's much better to lose weight at a slower, steadier rate, focusing on a plan you can live with for life. In the end, it's a true lifestyle change that's going to affect weight loss.

Is a flat stomach a realistic goal?

Most women have a typical "pear" figure, while most men have the "apple" shape body type. I, however, was blessed with an apple figure – you know skinny legs with all weight gathering around my middle. I actually was teased because of my "stick legs" while my girlfriend, who had a pear figure, got taunts of "thunder thighs". We couldn't win.

But she does win when it comes to the healthier figure. The extra fat I carry around my midsection is harder on my heart than the weight on her legs.

On top of my shape, I am only 5'4" so the distance between my hip bone and rib cage is less than an inch – that's not much room for all my organs. So for years I tried to attain a flat stomach. And as you can imagine I failed.

A perfectly flat midsection is simply not a realistic goal for many people (including me). Even if you are very thin, your internal organs may give a slight roundness there. Other reasons that your stomach may not be as flat as you like include fluctuating hormones, water retention, and PMS. Abdominal bloating caused by digestive problems is a problem for many. Constipation, gas, and food intolerance are all associated with bloat.

Abdominal exercises can tighten and strengthen your stomach, but they won't reduce the layer of fat that is on top. When you lose weight, it happens all over the body. Spot reduction is a myth.

So don't get hung up on having a flat stomach. It's just not a realistic goal.

How can I maintain a normal resting heart rate?

Most of the time, you're probably unaware of your heart's activity—nearly 100,000 beats per day, or about 37 million beats per year. But have you ever been startled out of a sound sleep? Your heart is pumping so wildly you can actually feel it through your pajamas?

That's not a good time to take your heart rate. A good time to measure your heart rate is when you've been at rest. And take the measurement at your wrist not your neck. Remember to not use your thumb as it has a pulse of its own. To find your resting heart rate, press the index and middle fingers over the underside of the opposite wrist, just below the thumb. Press down gently until you feel your pulse. Count the beats for 15 seconds and then multiply by 4 for the total number of beats per minute.

A normal resting heart rate can vary from as low as 40 beats per minute (bpm) to as high as 100 bpm. But for women, we have an average of 75 bpm. Generally, a lower heart rate at rest implies more efficient heart function and better cardiovascular fitness.

Some people assume that if their heart rate is normal, their blood pressure must be normal too. Don't make that mistake. Heart rate and blood pressure are not the same. The only way to know your blood pressure is to measure it with a blood pressure cuff.

A resting heart rate higher than 80 beats per minute can be associated with a greater risk of becoming obese or developing heart disease later. Diabetes and obesity are both risky for the heart.

Stress can spike your resting heart rate, sometimes to beat more than 100 times per minute. Smoking or drinking a lot of caffeine can also do it. As well as dehydration, fever, anemia, and thyroid disease.

To improve your heart rate you can quit smoking, reduce caffeine intake, and drink enough water. One of the best ways to improve your heart rate is through exercise. The heart is a muscle, and, like all muscles, it grows stronger with exercise. The stronger it is, the more efficient it is, taking fewer beats to pump blood throughout the body.

What's the best way to reduce stress?

Many years ago, my dad suffered a heart attack, I sold my home, moved to a different city, and started my own small business. Talk about a stressful year. Besides the emotional feelings tied to the stress, my body's natural response to stress was to tense up.

Stress affects our body, and it's important to learn how to recognize when your stress levels are out of control. Typical physical symptoms include body aches and pains, diarrhea or constipation, nausea, dizziness, rapid heartbeat, and frequent colds. You can better cope with the physical symptoms of stress by strengthening your physical health. For example, set aside time to relax. Relaxation techniques such as meditation, prayer, and deep breathing activate the body's relaxation response, a state of restfulness that is the opposite of the stress response.

Also, exercise regularly. Physical activity plays a key role in reducing and preventing the effects of stress. Nothing beats aerobic exercise for releasing pent-up stress and tension. I ALWAYS feel better after I go for a walk.

Eat a healthy diet. Well-nourished bodies are better prepared to cope with stress. Start your day with a healthy breakfast and reduce your caffeine and sugar intake.

Get plenty of sleep. Feeling tired can increase stress by causing you to think irrationally. Keep your cool by getting a good night's sleep. And I'm a personal fan of a good afternoon nap.

My body's natural response to the stress those years ago was to tense up. To counter this, I would physically hike my shoulders up to my ears and then let them down slowly, imagining they had weights on them. This simple action relieved my shoulder stress relaxing my shoulders down to normal. Be aware of your body's specific response to stress and incorporate simple strategies to strengthen your physical health.

Are electronic stimulation devices good?

Have you ever found yourself up in the middle of the night, unable to sleep so you turned on the television and started to watch the shopping channel? Inevitably some fancy gadget comes on that you think, "I must have that." I hope if you fell victim to the night time buy-a-thon and pulled out your credit card to buy a cheesy product that you settled for something simple like a Ginsu Knife or ShamWow and not an electronic stimulation device. Manufacturers of these devices claim that these are equivalent to doing hundreds of exercises like sit-ups. But (as I'm sure you've heard) if it's too good to be true than it's probably not true.

Electrical stimulators work similarly to the nervous system—an electrical signal causes a specific muscle to contract. A key difference is that the body generates signals internally, while electrical stimulators generate the signal outside of the body. But the devices are not without risk.

Muscle injury, such as tears, can be caused by electrical muscle stimulation if the tissue becomes too tense during the electrically induced contraction. Pre-existing muscle injuries, such as tears and deep bruises, can get worse and may even prevent full tissue healing. Even skin can become irritated because of a reaction to the electrode adhesive or the electrical current itself. Those with pacemakers or implanted defibrillators are at much higher risk of shock.

No device develops a better body without any work on your part. There is no substitute for your own effort. If you want strong abdominal muscles without doing hundreds of sit-ups, you'd be better off taking a 30-day Plank Challenge to improve your core than spending oodles of money on a device that's potentially dangerous. So, next time you can't sleep stay away from the infomercials.

Are sauna suits good for weight loss?

Sauna suits, plastic wraps, rubber jumpsuits oh my! These are 3 things that make me want to cry.

Outrageous, outlandish, and potentially dangerous. Stay away from them. These suits are usually made of a material like nylon, plastic or rubberized vinyl that holds in body heat, causing sweating. The perspiring leads to dehydration and a temporary body-water weight loss.

Overheating is not only useless for permanent weight loss but also dangerous. Because of losing too much water too quickly, a person may experience symptoms related to heat stroke. Potential health risks include dehydration, weakness, dizziness, fainting and muscle cramps. Extended use of sauna suits for the purposes of quick weight loss can lead to serious health emergencies including organ failure due to extreme loss of electrolytes and even death related to heat stroke.

There is no evidence that suggests that wearing a sauna suit will increase the rate at which the body metabolizes body fat or that exercisers can expect long term benefits from continued use.

And if you've ever watch the National Lampoon's Christmas Vacation you'll catch a glimpse of Clark Griswold's neighbours coming in from a workout wearing silver suits. It's not only dangerous but it's hideously ugly.

There is simply no short cut to weight loss.

How do I buy the right shoes?

My shoe size used to be a 7. Now it's an 8. I blame my children. I believe that my kids caused my hips to widen, my height to shorten, and my feet to grow. Don't ask me how– it's just what I believe.

And I believe that my feet swell over the course of a day. This is, in fact, a proven phenomenon. So although conventional wisdom claims that the early bird gets the worm, it's actually not a good idea to buy shoes early in the day. You'll get a more comfortable fit if you buy shoes when your feet are at their largest. You're better off to go late in the day because your feet naturally swell as the day progresses.

And when you go to buy shoes go prepared. If you have special shoe inserts or orthotics, bring them along. If you're buying tennis shoes, don't try them on sockless or with dress socks. Wear socks exactly like those you'd wear during the particular sport you're playing.

Which brings me to my second point. Buy the right shoe to match the sport. I once bought running shoes and then wore them to an aerobics class. Keeping in mind that I'm not very coordinated to start the shoes really didn't help. They were designed for forward movement, not the side-to-side support that I needed for the class. Needless to say I had to dish out more money for a new pair of shoes that provided the cushioning and support.

Lastly, keep in mind that if the shoe doesn't feel right, don't buy it. A shoe that doesn't fit right in the store won't fit right down the road.

Is skipping breakfast a good way to lose weight?

As soon as I awake in the morning, my thoughts turn to breakfast. I'm a diehard cereal lover and I usually go over in my mind the choices I have in the cupboard. I actually can't even enjoy a coffee before I have some food in my belly. Breakfast has never been a problem for me.

But I know many people who cringe at the thought of eating anything before noon. They believe that skipping breakfast is a good way to lose weight.

But nothing could be further from the truth. In addition to missing nutrients and energy, it'll reduce your concentration and if you eat nothing at breakfast you can become ravenous and overeat the rest of the day.

Eating breakfast is one of the most efficient ways to get your body off to a good start. It is literally "breaking the fast" of the night before and provides you with the energy to start your day.

Choosing something simple like a banana and a yoghurt, or toast with peanut butter or even drinking a nutrient rich supplement or DIY smoothie would be better than nothing at all.

And Tony the Tiger agrees about the benefits of eating breakfast, "They're not good. They're Gr-r-reat!"

Will lifting weights make women bulk up?

One of my favourite haunts is Chapters bookstore. I love nothing more than to order a steamed milk at Starbucks and then browse through the books for hours on end. Sometimes I'll peruse the magazine rack and I'm often amazed at the variety of magazines available for every hobby, interest, and sport. I tend to migrate towards the fitness magazines with the body builders on the front cover. Muscles bulging over muscles. And it's not limited to men either. Women can have bulging muscles too.

But not the average woman. We just don't have the genetic makeup to develop huge muscles. The women on the covers of these magazines devote hours and hours a day lifting very heavy weights. They are on a specific diet and exercise regime to get that big.

So no worries if you think that by lifting weights you'll bulk up. This simply isn't true. Women have less of the hormone needed to build muscle bulk easily. And because muscle tissue is more dense than fat, adding a little bit more muscle to your body and decreasing your fat actually makes you look leaner—not bigger.

It'll not only help you lose weight, but you'll sleep better, have more energy, reduce your risk of heart disease, combat loss of bone and decrease your risk of osteoporosis.

So put your fears aside and start strength training today.

Can I exercise during sickness?

Cold and flu season can wreak havoc on your fitness program. My girlfriend recently suffered from a bout of the flu. She was coughing, felt achy and tired, and had nausea. She desperately wanted to continue with her exercise program but wisely decided to take some time off.

When your body is trying to fight an illness you don't want to overtax it with strenuous exercise because you could run the risk of getting even sicker. If you have a fever, exercising is a no-no.

However, with other symptoms it's not always easy to gauge whether you're too sick to exercise or not. If you have a cold, exercising may help you feel slightly better. A brisk walk can unclog your sinuses better than spending an afternoon on the couch. And gentle exercise will improve your circulation to help offset that listless, rundown feeling. Do what you can do and if you can't do it than don't.

But if you don't know if you should exercise or not do a "neck check". That is, if your symptoms are above the neck like sneezing, sore throat, tearing eyes, and runny nose then it's probably okay to work out.

If your symptoms are below the neck like my friend's coughing, body aches and fatigue, then wait until the symptoms subside.

Once you're feeling better, use shorter, less intense sessions to build slowly back up to your former level. When my friend was feeling less sickly, she started back with a walk instead of her usual run. As her body healed she increased her intensity until she was back up to her normal level.

Is eating two meals a day better for weight loss?

I remember a few years back when my husband and I took a vacation. It was wonderful to get away and enjoy the new sites and beauty of the land. But we found it was quite expensive. So we decided to buy only two meals a day instead of our usual three.

Although we saved in the cost of dining, I found myself eating more at those two meals than I would if I had eaten my customary three and still feeling hungry between sittings.

Skipping meals has a way of backfiring, especially if you're trying to lose weight. Like I did, you may become over hungry and over eat. Skipping just one meal causes your blood-sugar levels to dive and without a new supply of calories, your system shifts into starvation mode in an effort to conserve energy. Your metabolism slows, so the food you do eventually take in isn't burned off as efficiently.

You may want to eat several mini-meals of 400 calories (called grazing), instead of two meals of 1200 calories. It may feel counter intuitive to eat all day, but grazing helps to increase your energy, it can add variety to your diet, and it'll help you maintain your weight. Frequent snacking, as long as it's healthy keeps hunger at bay, and helps control blood sugar.

However, if you want to eat more often, be careful to keep your calories in check. Don't eat too much. Avoid processed foods, refined carbohydrates, and sugary drinks. Instead, fuel up on protein and high-fiber carbs. For example, raw veggies with ¼ cup of hummus for dipping.

Why not try grazing? Just watch the quality, calories, and portion sizes of your mini meals.

Is no gain without pain true?

With a last name like Payne it seemed only natural for me to become a personal trainer – No Gain without Payne, right?

Well, I think we know that although the slogan is popular it's not right. Exercise is not supposed to hurt.

While a little soreness is normal after you start exercising, pain isn't.

Like today, I can feel my inner thighs – they're a little sore. That's normal DOMS – delayed onset muscle soreness—from my lunges I did yesterday. But it's only mild discomfort not outright pain. When we exercise, the muscle produces a force to stretch the fibers which causes tiny tears in them. The soreness comes from the body repairing these fibers and building the muscle.

However, if pain is sharp or happens suddenly during your workout, it could mean you've actually injured yourself. Any pain experienced, whether during cardiovascular activity, strength training or stretching, is your body's way to warn you to stop what you're doing.

For the normal soreness of a workout it's good to take a rest, soak your muscles in a warm tub of Epsom salts, use anti-inflammatory medication, have a massage, and stretch.

Remember that muscle soreness can actually be encouraging as it gives you the signal that you are making forward strides in your health.

Can I still exercise after an injury?

Do you remember years ago the American gymnast who performed the vault in the 1996 Olympics despite having injured her ankle and she had to be carried to the podium by her coach?

Amazing, commendable, spectacular. But not recommended.

If you hurt yourself it's best to not continue working out.

Well actually you can still workout after an injury if you modify your workout to exercise around the injury.

For example, if you hurt your ankle or knee it wouldn't be a good idea to jog on it, but you may still be able to do other light exercises in a pool, or try a hand-bike, or even a stationary bike. If you are weight training, you may be able to train using lighter weights and higher repetitions. And whether it's a cardiovascular workout or a strength training workout make sure that you are warming up your muscles and stretching properly.

Also, don't forget nutrition. You can accelerate the healing process by getting adequate nutrition. Eat foods that are high in omega-3 fatty acids like flaxseed and fish, and anti-oxidants like grapes and blueberries.

Whatever you do, don't give up completely. Do what you can to help recover faster and stay on the road to health.

Do I need to add extra protein when I exercise?

I visited the local health food store to buy some groceries and happened to notice an entire wall full of high-protein powders, drinks, tablets, capsules and bars.

It's a booming business but not one I'm involved in. You might think that as an experienced personal trainer I would have recommended clients add extra protein to their diet. But I didn't.

The clients I worked with were average, regular people who were interested in improving health and maybe even losing a few pounds along the way. These people generally got enough protein in their diet. Feeding them more protein than they needed wouldn't help. As a matter of fact excess protein is converted to energy and then it's either burned up or stored as fat.

A research study published in the Journal of the American Medical Association determined that the optimal intake of protein for those 18 years of age and older was 0.8 g of protein per kilogram body weight per day. In plain English, this means .36 grams per pound of body weight or for a 140-pound woman that's about 50 grams. You can easily get this amount in your daily diet from Greek yogurt, eggs, chicken, tuna, and mixed nuts.

Now if you're an elite athlete or strength-trainer you will need more protein due to the simple fact their bodies are being "abused." The amount of protein for athletes should be at least .55 grams per pound per day. Depending upon your sport or training regimen, the daily requirement can even go as high as 1 gram/pound.

Protein is essential for growth and repair of muscles, bone, tendons, skin, hair, and other tissues.

But unless you're training for a marathon or entering a body building contest you most likely don't need to add a lot of high-protein, high cost, powdered drinks or bars to your diet.

Can I strength train without equipment?

I remember when I worked as a personal trainer and I had an elderly woman as a client. She was a retired teacher who lived alone in a small but comfortable home. She had never lifted weights before and she had no desire to get a gym membership but she wanted me to set her up on a strength training program.

No problem I thought. There are a number of ordinary floor exercises that I could show her that work with her own body weight for a complete muscle workout. Bodyweight exercises are a simple, effective way to improve balance, flexibility, and strength without machinery or extra equipment.

We started on her stairs and walked up and down, holding onto the handrail for balance. This helped get her blood moving and her heart rate up.

Looking around her living room, we decided to use her piano bench for back one-arm pull and tricep exercises.

In her kitchen we used the countertop as support for leg exercises such as side raises and calf lifts.

The hallway provided a clear wall for pushups and wall squats.

Since there's no equipment involved, bodyweight workouts make it easy to transition quickly from one exercise to the next. Shorter rest times mean it's easy to quickly boost heart rate and burn some serious calories.

Although my client was a beginner to exercising, bodyweight exercises are a great choice because they're easily modified to challenge any fitness level. They also are good to stave off boredom by adding extra repetitions, performing the exercises faster or super-slow and can even the simplest exercise more challenging.

So there really are no excuses for not exercising. Ask someone why they don't exercise, and chances are "no time" or "inconvenience" might come up as culprits.

Bodyweight exercises allow anyone to squeeze in workouts wherever they are.

You don't need a gym membership, or a block of hours to exercises. You can start today.

Is there such a thing as exercising too much?

Recently, I read a personal blog from a woman I admire. She wrote with transparency and honesty about her struggles especially over the last year. She shared that although she enjoyed her running schedule and training for marathons her body was telling her that she was exercising too much.

Thirty minutes a day of moderate physical activity is enough to help prevent things like diabetes, high cholesterol, and high blood pressure. But too much exercise can lead to injuries, exhaustion, depression, and suicide. It can also cause lasting physical harm. Your adrenal gland, pumping out hormones as you pound the pavement, can only produce so much cortisol at a time.

Just as exercising too little is not healthy, exercising too much is detrimental to your health as well.

It can compromise your immune system and increase your risk of injury.

The Journal of the American College of Cardiology researchers from Denmark say that people who push their bodies too hard may essentially undo the benefit of exercise. Those who ran at a fast pace more than four hours a week for more than three days a week had about the same risk of dying during the study's 12-year follow up as those who were sedentary and hardly exercised at all.

It's a good idea to take one full day a week to recover with little activity. The body needs a day of rest, especially if you are just starting out. And remember if you want to do something good for yourself, you don't have to be extreme.

Should I take vitamin supplements?

I remember learning years ago that Vitamin C was good to fight colds. So I bought chewable tablets and starting popping them like candy.

But then I learned that any excess vitamin C may cause nausea, diarrhea and stomach cramps, and your system will just flush it out. Money down the toilet – literally.

Vitamins are organic compounds needed in small quantities to sustain life. But we normally get the necessary amount from our daily diet, so I returned to getting my vitamin C from oranges and other citrus fruits, berries, and vegetables such as sweet red peppers and broccoli.

I've learned that a well-balanced diet is the best way to get the nutrients I need to stay healthy.

Pills and supplements should not take the role that is better delegated to food. They are supposed to "supplement" our diets. Food contains thousands of phytochemicals, fiber, and more that work together to promote good health that can't be duplicated with a pill or a cocktail of supplements.

Looking for Vitamin A? The highest concentration of vitamin A is found in sweet potatoes. B12? Vitamin B12 occurs naturally in beef liver, trout, salmon, and tuna. Calcium? Plain yogurt and dark, leafy greens.

Vitamin D? Fatty fishes (like salmon and mackerel) are among the few naturally occurring dietary sources of vitamin D.

We could go through the entire alphabet of vitamins and provide lots of delicious foods that provide these vitamins. The best place to get your vitamins is from your diet.

Is it possible to spot reduce fat?

Have you ever stood in front of a mirror and said something like, "If I could just take the fat from over here and move it up here?" Or even better just lose weight in a specific area of your body?

Oh, if it were only that easy. But unfortunately there is no diet or exercise program that is going to take the fat off of any particular area of your body.

You can reduce overall body fat, but you can't selectively take fat off a specific area of your body.

For example, a woman may have a lot of fat stored on her sides above the hips ("love handles") so she uses side-bend and abdominal side-to-side twisting exercises in an attempt to reduce those fat cells. But performing those exercises may strengthen the muscles responsible for those movements, but they have little impact on reducing the amount of fat stored there.

So, if you're doing a million sets of crunches and other ab exercises thinking it's having any direct effect whatsoever on the fat on your stomach... you are completely wasting your time. If anything, all you're doing is overtraining your abdominal muscles. The fat covering them will remain completely unchanged.

Can ankle weights help burn more calories?

Sometimes in our attempts to save time or work out more efficiently we try to combine two healthy activities into one. But this doesn't always work well and sometimes can even be dangerous.

For example, we may try to combine the healthy activity of walking with the healthy activity of lifting weights by putting weights on our wrists or ankles as we walk, thinking this will burn more calories.

Ankle weights and wrist weights come in the form of bands or pouches that have weights, sand or water inside. When strapped to your ankles or wrists, they add between three and 20 pounds of resistance to any lower and upper body movement.

However, walking with ankle weights can increase risk of injury to your knees, ankles and feet.

You could develop hip problems and shin splints. You might change your gait to accommodate the weights. Walking in an unnatural way could cause problems, straining and stressing other body parts as they compensate for the changed walking pattern.

Instead of wearing ankle weights when you walk, increase your speed; maybe jog for some of the time and walk for the rest. You could also climb hills to give yourself a better workout without wearing ankle weights. And if you really want to wear ankle weights wear them when you do leg raises with a machine at the gym.

As for energy expended, health experts say wrist weights may increase the amount of calories burned during an aerobic exercise. However, they also caution that these weights increase the workload on your joints. The heavier the weights on your wrists, the more burden on your wrists, elbows and shoulders.

This may, in turn, increase the likelihood of injuries like sprains, dislocations and ligament tears. Frequent users may also risk tendinitis, as this, too, is a condition that occurs as a result of frequent strain on your joints. Wrist weights can cause shoulder and elbow injuries.

This adds stress to the body in a way that it was not designed to handle, and the increased calorie burn is negligible.

What is a realistic weight loss goal?

A neighbour friend of mine told me that she'd lost 50 pounds. When I asked her how she'd done it, she said, "Very slowly."

She lost an average of one pound a week for 50 weeks. It took her almost a full year to take the weight off but the good news was that she was keeping it off. She committed to making simple changes. For example, she used to drink coffee with 2 scoops of sugar so she reduced it to one scoop. And she used to order a donut with her coffee but she vowed to quit that habit.

Losing something like 5 pounds a week isn't a realistic weight loss goal. If you lose weight too fast, chances are you'll gain it right back. Also, if you lose a lot of weight very quickly, you may not lose as much fat as you would with a more modest rate of weight loss. Instead, you might lose water weight or even lean tissue, since it's hard to burn that many fat calories in a short period.

An eating plan that's too restrictive doesn't meet your nutritional needs and you'll lose muscle along with fat. Very-low-calorie diets that result in rapid weight loss are often dangerously low in essential nutrients, including vitamins and minerals. A lack of vitamins can lead to a host of health problems, including immune system suppression and bad skin, hair and nails. Chronic mineral deficiencies may also have long-term effects on your health. A lack of essential minerals can lead to fluid imbalances, cardiac arrhythmia or an irregular heartbeat, muscle cramps and loss of bone mass.

Losing one pound a week is more realistic, and results in long-term weight loss if combined with exercise. Efforts are usually healthy and you'll probably maintain as permanent lifestyle changes.

Remember the fact that it may have taken you years to gain weight, so it's not a good idea to lose weight too quickly by over exercising or following very-low-calorie or crash diets. Crash diets may result in rapid initial weight loss but may have a negative effect on long-term health and diet compliance.

The slower the weight comes off the less likely it will come back.

Slow and steady is the name of the game when you're trying to lose weight.

Are fresh fruits more nutritious than frozen?

In 2013, I had the fantastic opportunity to visit Israel with my mom and a group of Christians from Ontario. There were many highlights but one of my fond memories was the food. We feasted on fresh fruits and vegetables every day. I especially enjoyed the citrus fruits like oranges and grapefruits. They were so fresh and packed with flavour.

Given a choice I prefer fresh fruits and vegetables over frozen. I love to buy my produce in the summer at roadside stands by local farmers. However, living in Canada limits the types of fruits and veggies that we can grow. So I'm happy to have my local grocery store to shop at.

But did you know that because frozen foods are generally sealed right away, nutrients are locked in and so they can actually be more nutritious than fresh produce?

Frozen fruit and vegetables can be healthier, with higher levels of vitamins and cancer fighting antioxidants, than leafy 'fresh' produce. Produce that's been hauled a long distance may lose nutrients on the trip, in storage, and sitting on the grocery store shelves. Fruits and vegetables chosen for freezing tend to be processed at their peak ripeness, a time when—as a general rule—they are most nutrient-packed.

While canned vegetables tend to lose a lot of nutrients during the preservation process (notable exceptions include tomatoes and pumpkin), frozen vegetables may be even more healthful than some of the fresh produce sold in supermarkets. When vegetables are in-season, buy them fresh and ripe. "Off-season," frozen vegetables will give you a high concentration of nutrients.

Does late night eating cause weight gain?

My mom challenged me to stop eating by 7 p.m. every night for 3 months. Both of us wanted to shed the extra weight we had added over the holidays. I accepted her challenge and took it one step further and created a "No Eating After 7 p.m." Facebook Group page. This group offered support and encouragement to stop the late night snacking.

But it's really a myth that you gain weight by eating late at night. The time of day you eat calories won't affect your weight. As long as you eat the same number of calories and maintain the same activity level over a 24-hour period, it doesn't matter what time it says on the clock.

The American Dietetic Association agrees and emphasizes that it's not the timing but the amount being eaten that can cause weight gain.

But there's the kicker. If you're like me, you eat a reasonable breakfast, lunch and supper but in the evenings, whether chilling out in front of the TV, visiting with a friend, or working late on your computer you munch, not because you're actually hungry but because you're tired, bored, stressed or socializing. You mindlessly eat high-calorie foods like chips, cookies, and candies and it's easy to eat the entire bag before you realize it.

Besides those unnecessary extra calories, eating too close to bedtime can cause indigestion and sleeping problems too.

It's okay to eat supper after 7 p.m. but after you've put away the dishes, vow to stay out of the kitchen and out of the chip bag.

Can food labels be trusted?

After 4 years of university, I graduated with a Bachelor Degree in Business. One of my favourite courses was marketing and I especially enjoyed the subject of advertising. Zig Ziglar was a creative master and I learned all kinds of fun and interesting ways that companies market and package their products.

But some of their marketing tactics bordered on unethical. Did you know that the word "Light" spelled "Light" or "Lite" on a food label doesn't necessarily mean it's low in calories or fat? The label could be referring to its colour or even its texture.

"Made with" doesn't naturally mean it's a good source of the ingredient. All it means is that it contains at least a bit of the ingredient. But since the label isn't defined by the FDA, we can't be sure how much it actually contains.

This is why we have the caveat "Buyer Beware". Don't be swayed by claims on the front of the package.

It's up to us, as the buyer, to read the nutritional panel for fat content and number of calories. And while you're looking keep an eye on fiber, sugar, and sodium as well. We want high fiber and low sugar and sodium.

Also have a look at the ingredient list. Remember that the closer an item is to the beginning of the list, the more of it the food contains. And the fewer the ingredients, the less processed the food generally is.

To beat the confusion? Buy the majority of your products at the grocery store without labels at all, such as fresh fruits, vegetables and lean meats.

Is fruit juice good for me?

Years ago, I joined Weight Watchers to help me with my over-eating. I liked their plan as they focused on healthy food choices, moderation, and they even recommended exercise.

One new thing that I discovered about my habits was that I drank many of my calories. I tended to drink a lot of apple and orange juice and counted it toward my daily fruit requirement.

However, it's better to get your nutrients from the actual fruit than to drink the juice. Fruit juice is loaded with sugar.

In fact, fruit juice contains as much sugar and calories as a soft drink.

It's also absorbed very fast, so by the time it gets to your stomach your body doesn't know whether it's Coca-Cola or orange juice. The British Medical Journal published a study which found fruit juice to be associated with an increased risk of type 2 diabetes.

While whole fruit is a source of dietary fiber, fruit juice actually contains little to no fiber. Juice can also be extremely easy to over-consume, which may take you over your recommended daily calorie intake.

So choose the whole fruit over fruit juice or as the adage says, "An apple a day keeps the doctor away."

How can I curb the mid-afternoon slump?

I'm a big believer in taking a daily nap and love to have 10 to 20 minutes of undisturbed quiet time in the afternoon. I think the countries that promote an afternoon siesta are brilliant and have got it right.

Many of us suffer from the mid-afternoon slump and this is a time we may reach for a handful of chocolate covered peanuts or some other sugary snack. But not only is eating sugar to get more energy counter-productive your body is most likely not calling for more refined carbohydrates but rather the slump may be a sign that you're not drinking enough water.

Dehydration is a common cause of daytime fatigue, as well as headaches, irritability, decreased alertness and concentration.

Water boosts our energy and improves our concentration. So instead of reaching for a Snickers bar, opt for a tall glass of water. And you can also get your water from foods like watermelon, cucumbers and most other fruits and vegetables.

How to know if you're drinking enough water? Check your urine. It should be pale yellow.

Beat the mid-afternoon slump: stay hydrated.

Is strength training important for weight loss?

I remember working as a personal trainer and I had a client who wanted to lose 50 pounds. He had a healthy diet but because of a sedentary job he never exercised. He wanted me to set him up on an aggressive cardiovascular plan to reach his goal weight.

When I suggested that he include strength training he balked and said that he didn't want to start lifting weights until he was within 25 pounds of his ideal weight.

Being the professional I was I set him up on a cardiovascular plan that included weight lifting right from the get go.

I explained how strength training is the cornerstone of weight management.

By lifting weights he would build muscle. This extra muscle in turn boosts metabolism. This boosted metabolism helps to burn more calories even when he was at rest. Studies have proven that a strength training workout can burn calories for up to 12-48 hours after your training session. And ultimately he would lose fat and keep it off.

Strength training also protects joints and ligaments, increases bone density and prevents osteoporosis, improves balance and coordination, improves posture and boosts stamina.

I'm happy to report that he followed my advice and reached his weight loss goal.

Are carbs good or bad for me?

If you search the Internet for no-carb diets you'll discover reams and reams of diets proclaiming that cutting out carbohydrates is the answer to losing weight.

But by cutting out carbohydrates you deprive yourself of sufficient fiber, vitamins, minerals and antioxidants. And both your brain and your muscles need carbohydrates as their primary fuel.

So which one's right? What's the answer? Both!

It's found in the definition of carbohydrates. Not all carbs are created equal. Carbohydrates are sugars that come in 2 main forms – simple and complex. The difference between them is how quickly they're digested and absorbed along with their chemical structure.

Simple carbohydrates are those high-sugar foods that are the quickest source of energy and rapidly digested. They include table sugar, brown sugar, corn syrup, honey, maple syrup, jams, and candy. They raise your blood glucose levels quickly. Complex carbohydrates are rich in fiber and usually high in vitamins and minerals. They include green vegetables, whole grains, lentils and beans.

Since complex carbohydrates come from plant-based foods, we know that those foods also contain a ton of beneficial nutrients including vitamins, minerals and antioxidants. The fiber in fruit helps slow the digestion of carbs, which is why your blood sugar doesn't spike as much after eating fiber-filled fruit like it does when you gulp down a soda or candy bar. So the goal is to reduce your intake of simple carbs while at the same time increasing your intake of complex carbs.

Is sweating a good way to lose weight?

I come from a long line of sweaters. Not the kind where you knit but rather the kind where you drip. My mother sweats, my grandmother sweated, and I can probably assume my great-grandmother sweated too. It's in our genes.

Although we tend to drench our head and wrist bands when we workout, we don't actually burn any more calories than the non-sweater beside us.

Working out in a hotter place will increase sweating. Sweating is your body's way of cooling off. When you sweat you lose water and salts and so while it is true that a person's body weight can drop a number of pounds following a vigorous sweating session that weight is quickly recovered by drinking water.

According to the Military Fitness Center, excessive sweating has no useful purpose in weight loss.

Contrary to the claims of saunas and other heated-room therapies, sweating is not an adequate technique for weight loss. Dehydration doesn't count as weight loss.

It may also lead to a number of health problems such as heatstroke, extreme loss of electrolytes, kidney damage, and cardiovascular-related emergencies.

Don't worry whether you're a sweater or not, just get out there and have fun exercising.

Is running bad for my knees?

Although I've tried running in the past, I've never experienced the "runner's high" and have maintained the excuse that I don't like to run because it's bad for my knees and it'll cause arthritis.

However, running itself will not cause the arthritis. Arthritis is genetic. If you already have arthritis, and you have bone to bone contact and no cartilage in your knee, running will make it worse. If you're running and the pain becomes such that it alters the way you run, then you're probably doing more harm to your knees and should go see your doctor.

It's also known that heavier people are at higher risk for arthritis. For every pound of weight a person carries – whether it's in their body or they put it on in a backpack – they have four pounds on the knee when running. In other words, if you weigh 100 pounds, there are 400 pounds of force on the knee with each foot strike. But inherently, running is good and healthy for most people.

We know that weight-bearing exercise, including running, actually helps prevent osteoporosis and osteoarthritis. Repetitive weight bearing and motion are good for the joints, and running essentially does that. The compressive motion helps bring more fluid in your knees and keeps them moving.

There are many other factors that go into how running can affect your knees such as weight, body structure, shoe selection, and technique. So if you're starting a running program, you may want to start with a walking program first, then slowly progress to an easy running program paying attention to these other factors.

In addition to starting slowly, you may also want to combine running with bicycling or some other cross training. Your knees will thank you for it.

Can sleep help with weight loss?

I'm a sleeper. Ever since I was a small child my mother never had to tell me to go to bed. I'd put myself to bed early and sleep until the late morning hours. I can easily sleep for 10-12 hours straight.

On average, you need about 7.5 hours of quality sleep per night. If you're getting this already, another half hour won't help you lose weight, but did you know that if you are a five-hour sleeper and start to sleep for seven hours a night, you can start dropping weight.

Exactly how lack of sleep affects your ability to lose weight has a lot to do with our nightly hormones, your hunger and fullness hormones, including two called ghrelin and leptin. Ghrelin is the hormone that tells you when to eat. When you are sleep-deprived, you have more ghrelin. Leptin is the hormone that tells you to stop eating. When you are sleep deprived, you have less leptin. More ghrelin plus less leptin equals weight gain.

Also, when you're short on sleep, it's easy to reach for a large latte to get moving and go for a chocolate bar or other comfort foods because you lack the impulse control to say no. You might be tempted to skip exercise because you're too tired, get takeout for dinner, and then turn in late because you're uncomfortably full.

There are three easy things you can do to help you get more sleep. The first is to avoid any caffeine in the afternoon because it will keep you in the lighter stages of sleep, which is associated with poorer sleep at night.

The second is to exercise during the day to help improve sleep quality. However, don't exercise too close to bedtime as it actually wakes you up.

And lastly, watch what you eat before bedtime. Stay away from a heavy, rich meal as it can increase risk of heartburn, which will certainly keep you up all night.

If you're trying to lose weight, have a look at your sleeping routine and try to make healthy changes.

As the mattress commercial says, Good Night and Sweet Dreams.

Do I need a sports bra?

I've often joked that the reason I'm not a runner is because I'd have to wear three bras. I've never quite found a good sports bra until I started to actually research what makes for the best support.

In buying a sports bra, I've learned 6 things to keep in mind. First, look for a bra that has separate cups instead of the uniboob compression kind. Since breast tissue moves in a figure-eight pattern when you run, walk, or jump, using a bra with cups will support you better.

Then, look for a sports bra that has special fabrics designed to support and wick away moisture. For maximum breathability, seek out sweat-wicking fabric with air holes, ideally under the breast and across the back.

Look for a sports bra with a band that doesn't move. It should fit snugly and comfortably. If you raise your hands above your head the band should not move. If it's up your rib cage, try a smaller band. If the bra has straps, try adjusting them.

Look for a sports bra with a proper cup size. There shouldn't be any bulging at the top or by the underarm. The cups shouldn't have any wrinkles or gaps. If the cup fabric is wrinkled, try a smaller size.

Lastly, look for a sports bra with comfortable straps. Many offer adjustable straps. Adjust them to feel supportive without digging into your shoulders.

It doesn't matter what size breasts you have, every woman experiences bouncing during physical activity.

Therefore, no matter what size you are, you should wear a sports bra while running or exercising.

Is swimming good for weight loss?

When I was 7 years old, my parents put in an inground pool. I grew up swimming and enjoyed many happy summers playing in the pool. But I never considered swimming good for weight loss. I always felt like eating a ton of food after I finished swimming.

However, I've since learned that because swimming requires every muscle in your body to work to keep you moving and staying afloat no other workout burns calories, boosts metabolism, and firms muscles in your body better than a swimming workout.
It's also kind to your body. Water basically neutralizes gravity, so you become virtually weightless when immersed, providing no stress to your joints.

On top of that it's been noted that a swimmer's blood pressure, cholesterol levels, cardiovascular performance, and cognitive functioning are all comparable to someone far younger.

That said, I think it's time for me to get back in the pool.

Is weight a good indication of health?

I had a friend who could eat whatever she wanted without gaining a pound. I used to marvel at how she could pack in a plate of French fries soaked in gravy and wash it down with a strawberry milkshake. Although she ate like this always and never exercised she weighed at least 20 pounds less than me – someone who watched what I ate and exercised daily.

But good health is more than a number on a scale.

Some doctors now think that the internal fat surrounding vital organs like the heart, liver or pancreas — invisible to the naked eye — could be as dangerous as the more obvious external fat that bulges underneath the skin.

The theory is that internal fat disrupts the body's communication systems. The fat surrounding internal organs might be sending the body mistaken chemical signals to store fat inside organs like the liver or pancreas. This could ultimately lead to insulin resistance, type 2 diabetes, or heart disease.

Good health includes lifestyle choices such as eating well, exercising regularly, managing stress, and treating risk factors for chronic disease. So, like my friend, a person may appear trim on the outside, but still carry too much fat and not enough muscle on the inside.

The key is what doctors and public health experts have been saying all along: get more exercise — whether you're thin or fat.

Can I gain muscle after age 40?

I recently celebrated my 47th birthday. Funny thing, I thought I was 47 all last year so I haven't really aged. But my body tells me otherwise.

As we age, our hormone levels decline and this is one reason we gain body fat and lose muscle. But you can still transform your body even if you are in your 40s, 50s or 60s. Don't fall into the trap of thinking your best years are behind you.

Just remember, as you age the body is more susceptible to injury. There are some things you need to keep in mind when strength training in your 40s and beyond:

Always warm up for at least 15 minutes before you lift weights. This increases your core temperature and helps the blood flow for the workout to come.

Use a combination of free weights and machines. As a youth your body is able to use a lot more free weight exercises but as you age your stabilizer muscles start to weaken which can leave your ligaments and tendons in danger of injury. Using machine lowers this risk.

Your exercise form and posture needs to perfect. Your body doesn't have the forgiveness of youth anymore so using poor form can easily result in injury.

Recovery time is a little longer so rest and recovery is critical; fewer days in the gym is going to be a must.

You can still gain muscle after 40 but your risk of injury may be a bit higher, your recovery and recuperation time may be slower, and in general you need to be smarter in how you train.

If you want to gain muscle you absolutely can. Just train smart. And this applies to any age.

Should women exercise differently than men?

When I first took an interest in strength training, I was a teenager in high school. I asked my older brother what to do and he set me up on a program much like his own. I, in turn, shared this routine with a boyfriend and we would occasionally lift weights together in the school gym.

Years later, as a personal trainer I set up the same programs for both women and men. For the most part, women can perform the same workouts as men.

However, because the female body is built differently—for example, women have softer ligaments and tendons and a much wider pelvis—exercises such as squats and lunges may need to be modified to ensure proper form.

Other than that there aren't many situations when women should train differently than men.

Obvious circumstances such as pregnancy would involve another discussion entirely. Aside from that, women should train like men with a program to build a powerful and beautiful body!

And remember, your choice of exercises depends on what you are training for, for life or for a particular sport. Everyone, regardless of gender should include a balance of cardio, strength, and flexibility exercises.

Are protein shakes good for weight loss?

My husband makes a protein shake every morning for breakfast. He mixes protein powder with strawberries, milk, flax seed oil, hemp seeds, and sometimes bananas. For me, he creates shakes with mango and I take it in a thermos to work. I drink it in lieu of a typical lunch, not in addition to it. I do this neither to build a more muscly physique nor to lose weight but rather for convenience.

If you're drinking protein shakes because you believe they'll build muscle, you're mistaken.

Sports dietician Greg Shaw, of the Australian Institute of Sport, says, "If you're just sucking down the shakes, that isn't going to help. You must do resistance exercises alongside taking the protein shakes."

Also, if you're drinking protein shakes to lose weight, you're mistaken. Since protein contains calories, consuming too much can actually make losing weight more difficult—especially if you drink protein shakes in addition to your usual diet, and you're not exercising.

Protein shakes can be tasty and loaded with healthy ingredients. But keep in mind that they should only be used to supplement a well-balanced diet, not replace it.

About the author

Kimberley Payne is a motivational speaker and writer. Her writing relates raising a family, pursuing a healthy lifestyle, and everyday experiences to building a relationship with God. Kimberley offers practical, guilt-free tips on improving spiritual and physical health. Visit her website www.kimberleypayne.com

Did you enjoy this book? Please take a moment to write a review and share the blessings.

Books in the Fit for Faith Series

Fit for Faith – 7 weeks to improved spiritual and physical health
Want to get on the road to a healthy body and spirit? Discover ways to balance the physical and spiritual.

Women of Strength – a devotional to improve spiritual and physical health
Need motivation to improve whole health? Explore these inspirational reflections, simple exercises and uplifting prayers.

Get the Skinny – Answers to 45 Frequently Asked Health & Fitness Questions
Have health, weight and fitness questions? Learn the answers to live healthier and happier lives.

JumpStart – A Catalyst to Launch you into a Daily Spiritual & Physical Health Routine
Want to make simple changes to improve spiritual and physical health? Discover a daily, specific program to create a routine.

Healthy Body, Healthy Spirit: 4 Key Habits to Improve Your Personal Health
Want to learn from the experts? Discover these four key habits to set your life.

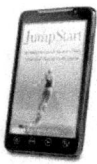 **Your Free Gift**

JumpStart – Launch your journey to improve physical and spiritual fitness

Want to make simple changes to improve spiritual and physical health? Discover a daily, specific program to create a routine.

Visit https://www.kimberleypayne.com/jumpstart/